OBEYSITY TO FIT

Everything you need to know about fitness and Lose 90 Pounds in 90 Days!

ACKNOWLWEDGEMENT

The fact that the author didn't begin her journey toward a healthier lifestyle until she was 42 years old gives the information in this book a unique perspective. At the age of 45, she was awarded a pro card to compete in the women's bikini division. The author, who is a nutritionist as well as a fitness and wellness coach, discusses the difficulties that a lot of individuals have when it comes to keeping a good diet and remaining physically fit as we get older.

The content of the book covers a wide variety of topics, some of which are as follows: how to meal prep for success

How to decide on a fitness center

Way to determine how much weight to carry.

How hormonal imbalances can impact one's ability to lose fat

The formulas for calculating calories and macronutrients

The book contains a variety of information that can be useful, such as a macro cheat sheet, an example meal prep menu, healthy food swaps, and fitness pictures. This book is for anyone of any age who has the desire to make improvements to their health and fitness but does not know where to start making those changes. In addition to this, many of the author's actual life experiences are included in the book. From her early years, during which she was raised on a farm in England, to more recent times, when she has been helping people learn about fat reduction and strength training via her many social media platforms, her life has been full of interesting experiences. Fluffy to Fit is a humorous and motivational fitness journey with the goal of showing you that you, too, are capable of achieving your fitness goals.

Table of Contents

CHAPTER 1

HOW IT ALL STARTED

Obesity is a complex condition that typically develops as a result of multiple factors, including genetics, lifestyle, and environmental influences. It doesn't have a single, straightforward cause, but rather arises from a combination of these factors. Here are some key factors that contribute to the development of obesity:

Genetics: Some people may have a genetic predisposition to obesity, meaning that their genes make them more likely to gain weight and store fat. However, genetics alone do not determine obesity; they interact with other factors.

Poor Diet: Consuming a diet high in calories, particularly from processed foods, sugary beverages, and high-fat foods, can contribute to weight gain. Overeating and regularly consuming more calories than the body needs can lead to obesity.

Lack of Physical Activity: A sedentary lifestyle, characterized by minimal physical activity and prolonged periods of sitting, can lead to weight gain and obesity. Regular physical activity is essential for burning calories and maintaining a healthy weight.

Environmental Factors: The modern environment often promotes obesity. Factors like easy access to unhealthy foods, larger portion sizes, and reduced opportunities for physical activity (e.g., due to desk jobs or urban environments that discourage walking) can contribute to obesity.

Psychological Factors: Emotional factors, such as stress, depression, and boredom, can lead to overeating and weight gain. People may use food as a way to cope with these emotions.

Obesity is a multifaceted condition influenced by a range of factors, including psychological factors.

Psychological factors can play a significant role in the development and management of obesity. Here are some key psychological factors associated with obesity:

1. **Emotional Eating:** Emotional factors, such as stress, anxiety, depression, and boredom, can lead to emotional eating. People may turn to food as a way to cope with difficult

emotions or as a source of comfort. This can result in overeating and weight gain.

2.   **Food Addiction:** Some individuals may develop an addiction-like relationship with certain foods, especially those high in sugar, salt, and unhealthy fats. Cravings and compulsive eating of these foods can contribute to obesity.

3.   **Body Image and Self-Esteem:** Poor body image and low self-esteem can contribute to disordered eating habits and a negative relationship with food. People with negative body image may engage in unhealthy dieting practices or have distorted perceptions of their bodies.

4.   **Binge Eating Disorder (BED):** BED is an eating disorder characterized by

recurrent episodes of overeating, often in response to emotional triggers. It can lead to significant weight gain and obesity.

5.   **Eating as a Coping Mechanism:** Some individuals may use food as a way to cope with life's challenges and stressors. Food may provide temporary relief or

distraction from emotional discomfort.

6. **Lack of Self-Control:** A lack of self-control or difficulty in regulating eating behavior can be a psychological factor contributing to obesity. This can manifest as impulsivity or a tendency to give in to cravings easily.

7. **Social and Environmental Influences:** Peer pressure, cultural

norms, and the availability of unhealthy foods in social settings can influence eating behaviors. People may eat more or make unhealthy choices in social situations, contributing to obesity.

8. **Childhood Experiences:** Adverse childhood experiences, such as trauma or neglect, can have long-lasting psychological effects that may contribute

to unhealthy eating patterns and obesity later in life.

9. **Mental Health Conditions:** Certain mental health conditions, such as bipolar disorder, schizophrenia, and some anxiety disorders, may be associated with weight gain due to the side effects of medications or disruptions in eating patterns.

10. **Stigma and Discrimination:** Experiencing weight-related stigma and discrimination can have profound psychological effects, leading to negative emotions, stress, and potentially worsening eating habits.

11. **Motivation and Goal Setting:** Motivation and the ability to set and work toward health-related goals

can play a positive role in obesity management. Psychological interventions that help individuals set achievable goals and maintain motivation can be beneficial.

It's important to note that these psychological factors often interact with other factors, such as genetics, environment, and lifestyle choices. Addressing the psychological aspects of obesity is a crucial component of obesity management and often involves therapies like cognitive-behavioral therapy (CBT), dialectical-behavior therapy (DBT), or counseling to help individuals develop healthier relationships with food, improve self-esteem, and learn more adaptive coping strategies for managing emotions. A holistic approach to obesity management considers both the physical and psychological aspects of the condition.

Socioeconomic Factors: Economic disparities can influence access to nutritious foods and opportunities for physical activity. Individuals with lower incomes may have limited access to healthy options and may rely more on inexpensive, calorie-dense foods.

Sleep Deprivation: Poor sleep patterns and inadequate sleep can disrupt hormonal regulation of appetite and increase cravings for unhealthy foods, contributing to weight gain.

Medications and Medical Conditions: Some medications can lead to weight gain as a side effect. Additionally, certain medical conditions, such as polycystic ovary syndrome (PCOS), hypothyroidism, and hormonal imbalances, can make it easier for individuals to gain weight.

Social and Cultural Factors: Social and cultural norms can influence eating behaviors and body image. For example, certain cultures may place a premium on larger body sizes, while others may emphasize thinness.

Childhood Obesity: Childhood obesity can set the stage for adult obesity. Children who are overweight or obese are more likely to continue carrying excess weight into adulthood.

It's important to note that obesity is a chronic condition that can have serious health consequences, including an increased risk of heart disease, diabetes, certain cancers, and other health problems. Preventing or managing obesity often requires a comprehensive approach that addresses these contributing factors through lifestyle changes, dietary modifications, increased physical activity, and, in some cases, medical interventions. If you are concerned about obesity or weight management, it is advisable to consult with a healthcare professional for personalized guidance and support.

CHAPTER 2

FOOD, GLORIOUS FOOD

While "Food, Glorious Food" from the musical "Oliver!" celebrates the joy of food, it's important to recognize that the health implications of food can vary widely depending on the choices we make. Food is essential for providing the body with the nutrients it needs to function properly and maintain good health. However, not all food is created equal, and the quality and quantity of what we consume can significantly impact our well-being. Here are some key points to consider regarding food and health:

1. **Nutrient Balance:** A healthy diet should include

a balance of essential nutrients such as carbohydrates, proteins, fats, vitamins, and minerals. These nutrients play critical roles in maintaining bodily functions, growth, and overall health.

2. **Whole Foods:** Whole, minimally processed foods like fruits, vegetables, whole grains, lean proteins, and healthy fats are

generally better choices for health. They are typically rich in nutrients and fiber and lower in added sugars, unhealthy fats, and artificial additives.

3.   **Portion Control:** Overeating and consuming large portions can contribute to weight gain and obesity. Paying attention to portion sizes is

important for maintaining a healthy weight.

4.   **Variety:** A varied diet ensures that you receive a wide range of nutrients. Eating a diverse selection of foods can also make meals more enjoyable and prevent dietary monotony.

5.   **Hydration:** Staying hydrated is crucial for good

health. Water is essential for digestion, circulation, temperature regulation, and overall well-being.

6.   **Limiting Processed Foods:** Highly processed foods, often high in sugar, unhealthy fats, and sodium, should be consumed in moderation. Excessive consumption of processed foods can lead to various health issues, including

heart disease, diabetes, and obesity.

7.   **Special Dietary Needs:** Some individuals may have specific dietary requirements due to allergies, intolerances, or medical conditions. It's important to tailor one's diet to meet these needs under the guidance of a healthcare professional or dietitian.

8. **Moderation:** Enjoying occasional treats or indulgent foods in moderation is a balanced approach to eating. It's okay to savor your favorite foods as part of an overall healthy diet.

9. **Mindful Eating:** Paying attention to hunger and fullness cues, eating slowly, and savoring each bite can

help prevent overeating and promote a healthier relationship with food.

10. **Consulting Professionals:** If you have specific dietary concerns or health conditions, it's advisable to consult with a registered dietitian or healthcare provider who can provide personalized guidance and recommendations.

In summary, while food can indeed be glorious and enjoyable, it's essential to make thoughtful choices that prioritize both taste and health. A well-balanced diet that includes a variety of nutrient-rich foods in appropriate portions is key to supporting overall health and well-being.

CHAPTER 3

HOW TO CALCULATE MACROS

Calculating macros, short for macronutrients, involves determining the appropriate amounts of carbohydrates, proteins, and fats you should consume in your daily diet based on your goals, such as weight loss, muscle gain, or maintenance. Here's a step-by-step guide on how to calculate macros:

1. Determine Your Goal:

- Are you looking to lose weight, gain muscle, or

maintain your current weight? Your goal will influence your macro ratios.

2. Calculate Your Total Daily Energy Expenditure (TDEE):

. Your TDEE is the number of calories you need to maintain your current weight. Several online calculators can help estimate your TDEE based on factors like age, gender, activity level, and weight.

3. Set Your Daily Caloric Intake:

- Depending on your goal, adjust your daily caloric intake:

  - Weight Loss: Create a calorie deficit by consuming fewer calories than your TDEE.

  - Weight Maintenance: Consume calories equal to your TDEE.

. Weight Gain (Muscle
Building): Create a
calorie surplus by
consuming more
calories than your TDEE.

4. Determine Your Macro Ratios:

. Macro ratios vary based on
your dietary preferences
and goals. Here are some
common ratios:

. Balanced: 40% carbs,
30% protein, 30% fat

- Low Carb: 10-30% carbs, 40-50% protein, 30-40% fat

- High Carb: 50-60% carbs, 15-25% protein, 15-25% fat

5. Calculate Your Macros:

- To calculate your macros, you'll need to convert your daily caloric intake into grams of each macronutrient, as each provides a different number of calories per gram:

- Carbohydrates: 4 calories per gram

- Proteins: 4 calories per gram

- Fats: 9 calories per gram

- For example, if you're following a balanced diet of 2,000 calories per day with a 40/30/30 macro ratio:

  - Carbohydrates: (40% of 2,000 calories) / 4

calories per gram = X
grams of carbs

- Proteins: (30% of 2,000
  calories) / 4 calories per
  gram = X grams of
  protein

- Fats: (30% of 2,000
  calories) / 9 calories per
  gram = X grams of fat

6. Adjust Based on Your Progress:

- Monitor your progress,
  such as changes in weight

and body composition, and adjust your macros as needed. You may need to fine-tune your ratios based on how your body responds to your current diet.

7. Track Your Food Intake:

. Use a food tracking app or journal to log your daily food intake to ensure you're meeting your macro goals.

8. Consult a Professional:

. For personalized guidance and to account for individual factors like medical conditions or dietary restrictions, consider consulting with a registered dietitian or nutritionist.

Remember that calculating macros is just one approach to managing your diet. It's essential to prioritize nutrient-dense foods and make healthy choices within your chosen macro ratios. Additionally, individual responses to macronutrient ratios can vary, so what works best for one person may not work for another. Be patient, stay consistent, and make adjustments as needed to reach your health and fitness goals.

CHAPTER 4

HOW TO CALCULATE CALORIES

Calculating calories involves determining the number of calories in the foods and beverages you consume as well as estimating your daily calorie needs for various purposes, such as weight maintenance, weight loss, or weight gain. Here's a guide on how to calculate calories:

1. Calculate Basal Metabolic Rate (BMR):

Your Basal Metabolic Rate (BMR) is the number of calories your body needs to maintain basic functions at rest. You can calculate your BMR using the Mifflin-St Jeor Equation:

For Men: BMR = (10 * weight in kg) + (6.25 * height in cm) - (5 * age in years) + 5

For Women: BMR = (10 * weight in kg) + (6.25 * height in cm) - (5 * age in years) - 161

2. Account for Activity Level (Total Daily Energy Expenditure - TDEE):

Your Total Daily Energy Expenditure (TDEE) includes not only your BMR but also the calories you burn through physical activity and the thermic effect of food (calories burned during digestion). To estimate your TDEE, multiply your BMR by an activity level multiplier:

- Sedentary (little to no exercise): BMR * 1.2

- Lightly active (light exercise or sports 1-3 days a week): BMR * 1.375

- Moderately active (moderate exercise or sports 3-5 days a week): BMR * 1.55

- Very active (hard exercise or sports 6-7 days a week): BMR * 1.725

- Super active (very hard exercise, physical job, or training twice a day): BMR * 1.9

3. Set Your Calorie Goal:

Depending on your goals, you can adjust your daily calorie intake:

- Weight Loss: Create a calorie deficit by consuming

fewer calories than your
TDEE. A common guideline
is to aim for a deficit of 500
to 1,000 calories per day,
which can result in a weight
loss of about 1 to 2 pounds
per week.

. Weight Maintenance:
Consume calories equal to
your TDEE to maintain your
current weight.

. Weight Gain: Create a
calorie surplus by
consuming more calories

than your TDEE. A surplus of 250 to 500 calories per day is often recommended for gradual and controlled weight gain.

4. Monitor Your Caloric Intake:

To calculate the calories in the foods you eat, you can use various resources, including food labels, nutritional databases, and mobile apps. Keep track of your daily calorie intake by recording what you eat and drink.

5. Adjust Based on Progress:

Regularly assess your progress and make adjustments as needed. If you're not achieving your desired results, you may need to modify your calorie intake.

6. Be Mindful of Nutrient Quality:

While calories are essential, it's equally important to consider the quality of the calories you consume. Focus on nutrient-dense foods that provide essential vitamins, minerals, and other nutrients along with calories.

7. Consult a Professional:

If you have specific dietary needs, health conditions, or unique goals, consider consulting with a registered dietitian or nutritionist. They can provide personalized guidance and meal plans.

Remember that accurate calorie calculation is a valuable tool for managing your weight, but individual variations and factors such as metabolism, genetics, and health conditions can impact your results. It's essential to approach calorie calculations as a starting point and adjust as necessary based on your unique circumstances and goals.

CHAPTER 5

MEAL PREP FOR SUCCESS

Meal prepping is a valuable strategy for achieving your nutritional goals, whether you're aiming to eat healthier, save time, or manage your portions more effectively. It involves preparing and portioning meals and snacks in advance, so they are readily available when you need them. Here's a guide on how to meal prep for success:

1. Set Clear Goals: Before you start meal prepping, define your goals. Are you looking to eat healthier, lose weight, save money, or simply have more convenient meals during the week? Having clear objectives will help you plan your meals effectively.

2. Plan Your Meals:

- Decide which meals you want to prep (e.g., breakfast, lunch, dinner, snacks) and for how many days. You can start with prepping just a few meals per week and gradually increase as you become more comfortable.

3. Create a Weekly Menu:

- Develop a menu for the week, including breakfast, lunch, dinner, and snacks. Incorporate a variety of foods to ensure a balanced diet with a mix of protein, carbohydrates, and healthy fats.

4. Make a Shopping List: Based on your menu, create a shopping list that includes all the ingredients you'll need for your meal prep. Stick to your list to avoid unnecessary purchases.

5. Set Aside Dedicated Time: Choose a specific day or time each week for meal prep.

Consistency is key to success. It might be Sunday afternoon or any other day that works for you.

6. Invest in Containers: Purchase a variety of containers in different sizes to accommodate your meals. Glass containers with lids are a popular choice because they are reusable and environmentally friendly.

7. Cook in Batches: Prepare your meals in large batches.

For example, you can cook a week's worth of chicken, rice, or vegetables at once. This saves time and ensures you have ingredients ready to assemble into meals.

8. Portion Control: Use kitchen scales or measuring cups to portion out your meals accurately. This helps manage calorie intake and ensures you're meeting your nutritional goals.

9. Label and Date: Label your containers with the date of preparation to keep track of freshness. Include any reheating instructions if necessary.

10. Include Variety: - Rotate your menu and ingredients to prevent meal fatigue. Explore new recipes and cuisines to keep things interesting.

11. Freeze for Later: - If you're prepping meals for more than a few days ahead, consider freezing some portions to maintain freshness. Just remember to label and date them.

12. Mindful Eating: - Even with meal prep, practice mindful eating. Pay attention to portion sizes, hunger cues, and your body's needs.

13. Be Flexible: - Life can be unpredictable. Be prepared to adjust your meal plan if your schedule changes or if you have unexpected events.

14. Stay Organized: - Keep your kitchen organized, and regularly clean out your fridge and pantry to avoid food waste.

15. Seek Support: - Share your meal prep journey with family or friends. Having a support system can make the process more enjoyable and hold you accountable.

Meal prepping can help you save time, money, and make healthier choices. It's a powerful tool for achieving your nutrition and wellness goals while maintaining a busy lifestyle. Remember that consistency and planning are essential for meal prep success.

Chapter 6

HOW TO DEAL WITH SUGAR CRAVINGS

Sugar cravings are common, and many people struggle with them. Excessive sugar consumption can have negative effects on health, including weight gain and an increased risk of chronic diseases. Learning how to manage and reduce sugar cravings is essential for maintaining a balanced and healthy diet. Here are strategies to help you deal with sugar cravings:

1. Identify Triggers:

- Pay attention to what triggers your sugar cravings. Is it stress, boredom, or certain situations? Identifying triggers can help you address the underlying causes of your cravings.

2. Gradual Reduction:

- Rather than quitting sugar abruptly, consider gradually reducing your sugar intake. This can make the transition easier and reduce withdrawal symptoms.

3. Choose Whole Foods:

- Opt for whole foods like fruits, vegetables, whole grains, and lean proteins. These foods are naturally sweet and can help satisfy your sweet tooth without the added sugars found in processed snacks and desserts.

4. Eat Regular Meals:

- Skipping meals or going too long between meals can lead to blood sugar fluctuations, which may trigger cravings. Eat balanced meals at regular intervals to stabilize blood sugar levels.

5. Stay Hydrated:

- Sometimes thirst can be mistaken for hunger or sugar cravings. Drink plenty of water throughout the day to stay hydrated.

6. Practice Mindful Eating:

- Slow down and pay attention to your food while eating. Mindful eating can help you savor the flavors and textures of your meals, making you less likely to crave sugary snacks.

7. Opt for Healthy Snacks:

. If you need a snack, choose healthier options like nuts, Greek yogurt, or sliced vegetables with hummus. These snacks provide nutrients and protein, helping you stay satisfied.

8. Avoid Highly Processed Foods:

. Highly processed foods often contain hidden sugars. Check food labels for ingredients like high fructose corn syrup, sucrose, or syrups, and limit your consumption of these products.

9. Plan Your Meals and Snacks:

- Plan your meals and snacks in advance to ensure you have nutritious options readily available. This can prevent impulsive choices that lead to sugar consumption.

10. Get Enough Sleep: - Lack of sleep can disrupt hunger hormones, making you more prone to cravings, including sugar. Aim for 7-9 hours of quality sleep per night.

11. Manage Stress: - Find healthy ways to manage stress, such as meditation, deep breathing exercises, yoga, or hobbies you enjoy. High stress levels can increase sugar cravings.

12. Consider Sugar Alternatives: - If you must satisfy a sugar craving, consider using natural sugar alternatives like stevia, erythritol, or monk fruit. These options can provide sweetness without the calories and potential negative effects of refined sugar.

13. Seek Support: - Share your goals with friends or family members who can support your efforts to reduce sugar intake. Having a support system can help you stay on track.

14. Professional Help: - If you find it challenging to control sugar cravings despite your best efforts, consider seeking guidance from a registered dietitian or healthcare professional who can provide personalized strategies and support.

Remember that managing sugar cravings is a process that

requires patience and persistence. It's okay to occasionally indulge in sugary treats, but the key is to do so in moderation and to build a healthy relationship with sweets over time.

CHAPTER 7

THE IMPORTANCE OF REST AND RECORVERY

Rest and recovery are essential components of a healthy and productive lifestyle. In today's fast-paced world, many people underestimate the significance of allowing their bodies and minds to rest and recuperate. However, adequate rest and recovery are crucial for physical, mental, and emotional well-being. Here, we explore the importance of rest and recovery:

1. Physical Recovery:

- **Muscle Repair:** Rest allows the body to repair and rebuild muscles that have been stressed during physical activities, such as exercise and sports.

- **Injury Prevention:** Adequate rest helps prevent overuse injuries and reduces the risk of accidents caused by fatigue.

- **Immune System Support:** Sleep and rest play a vital

role in strengthening the immune system, helping the body fight off illnesses and infections.

. **Hormonal Balance:** Restorative sleep and relaxation contribute to hormonal balance, including the regulation of cortisol (the stress hormone) and growth hormone.

2. Mental and Emotional Recovery:

- **Stress Reduction:** Rest and relaxation are effective in reducing stress levels and promoting mental clarity.

- **Emotional Resilience:** Adequate rest enhances emotional resilience, making it easier to cope with daily challenges and stressors.

- **Improved Concentration:** Restorative sleep and

breaks during the day
improve focus, memory,
and overall cognitive
function.

. **Enhanced Creativity:** Rest
provides the mental space
for creativity and problem-
solving, fostering
innovation and new ideas.

3. Sleep Quality:

. **Sleep Hygiene:** Proper rest
promotes good sleep
hygiene, which includes
establishing a consistent

sleep schedule, creating a comfortable sleep environment, and avoiding stimulants before bedtime.

- **REM Sleep:** Rapid Eye Movement (REM) sleep, which occurs during deep rest, is essential for emotional processing, memory consolidation, and learning.

4. Physical Performance:

- **Athletic Performance:** Athletes require sufficient

rest and recovery to optimize their physical performance, reduce the risk of injuries, and enhance muscle growth and adaptation.

- **Recovery Strategies:** Strategies such as stretching, foam rolling, and contrast baths can aid in post-workout recovery.

5. Long-Term Health:

- **Chronic Health Conditions:** Inadequate rest and

chronic sleep deprivation are associated with an increased risk of various health conditions, including obesity, heart disease, diabetes, and mood disorders.

6. Productivity and Creativity:

- **Efficiency:** Short breaks throughout the day can boost productivity by preventing burnout and fatigue, allowing you to return to tasks with renewed focus.

- **Problem-Solving:** Rest allows your mind to process information and fined innovative solutions to challenges.

7. Life Balance:

- **Social Connection:** Adequate rest ensures that you have the energy and mental clarity to maintain healthy social connections and relationships.

. **Self-Care:** Rest is a fundamental aspect of self-care. Prioritizing rest demonstrates self-compassion and a commitment to overall well-being.

In conclusion, rest and recovery are not signs of weakness but rather pillars of a healthy and fulfilling life. They enable you to perform at your best, both physically and mentally, while also safeguarding your long-term health. Incorporating regular periods of rest and adequate sleep into your routine is essential for achieving balance, resilience, and lasting vitality.

Chapter 8:

Cheat Meals, Not Cheat Days

Cheat meals and cheat days are terms often used in the context of diet and nutrition. While they can offer some psychological relief and flexibility within a diet plan, it's essential to approach them mindfully and avoid overindulgence. In this chapter, we'll discuss the concept of cheat meals and why moderation and balance are key:

Understanding Cheat Meals:

1.   What is a Cheat Meal?
A cheat meal is a planned deviation from your regular diet. It typically involves indulging in foods or dishes that you might avoid on your regular eating plan, often because they are high in calories, sugar, or unhealthy fats.

2.   Why Have Cheat Meals?
Cheat meals can serve several purposes:

- **Psychological Relief:** They can help satisfy cravings and reduce feelings of deprivation, making it easier to stick to a healthy eating plan.

- **Metabolic Benefits:** Occasional increases in calorie intake can boost metabolism and prevent it from slowing down due to prolonged calorie restriction.

3. **Portion Control:** The key to a successful cheat

meal is moderation. Instead of an entire cheat day, which can lead to excessive calorie intake, opt for a single meal where you indulge in a reasonable portion of your favorite treats.

Guidelines for Successful Cheat Meals:

1. **Plan in Advance:** Decide when and what your cheat meal will be. Planning helps you avoid impulsive, unhealthy choices.

2. **Set Limits:** Determine the portion size and the number of indulgent items you'll consume during your cheat meal.

3. **Enjoy Mindfully:** Savor every bite during your cheat meal. Eating slowly and mindfully can help you fully appreciate the flavors and prevent overeating.

4. **Balance with Nutritious Foods:** Surround your cheat meal with nutrient-dense foods.

For example, if you plan to enjoy a dessert, balance it with a salad or a lean protein source during your regular meals.

5.   **Stay Hydrated:** Drink plenty of water before and during your cheat meal to help control your appetite and prevent excessive calorie consumption.

Avoiding Cheat Day Pitfalls:

1.   **Overindulgence:** The term "cheat day" can lead to

excessive calorie intake and undermine your progress. It's easy to consume far more calories than you realize in a whole day of indulgence.

2.   **Guilt and Regret:** Overindulgence can lead to feelings of guilt and regret, which can negatively impact your relationship with food.

3.   **Binge Eating:** Cheat days sometimes lead to binge eating, where you

consume large quantities of
unhealthy foods in a short
period.

CHAPTER 9

ALCOHOL AND FAT LOSS

Alcohol is a common part of social gatherings and celebrations, but it can have implications for your fat loss goals and overall health. In this chapter, we'll explore the relationship between alcohol consumption and fat loss, and provide guidelines for making informed choices:

1. Calories in Alcohol:

Alcohol is calorie-dense, containing approximately 7 calories per gram, which is close to the calorie content of fat (9 calories per gram). While alcohol itself doesn't contain fat, the calories it provides can contribute to your daily calorie intake.

2. Alcohol and Fat Metabolism:

When you consume alcohol, your body prioritizes metabolizing it over other nutrients like carbohydrates, fats, and proteins. This can temporarily slow down the fat-burning process.

3. Impacts on Appetite and Food Choices:

Alcohol can lower inhibitions and impair judgment, which may lead to poor food choices and overeating when you're under the influence. Alcohol can also stimulate appetite.

4. Alcohol and Sleep:

Excessive alcohol consumption can disrupt sleep patterns, which can negatively impact fat loss efforts. Poor sleep can lead to increased cravings for unhealthy foods and reduced motivation for physical activity.

5. Alcohol and Muscle Recovery:

Alcohol can hinder muscle recovery and growth, as it can interfere with protein synthesis and impair nutrient absorption.

6. Guidelines for Alcohol Consumption During Fat Loss:

If you choose to include alcohol in your diet while pursuing fat loss, here are some guidelines to consider:

- **Moderation:** Consume alcohol in moderation. Guidelines for moderate drinking typically suggest up to one drink per day for women and up to two drinks per day for men. This is defined as:

- 12 ounces of beer (with about 5% alcohol content)

- 5 ounces of wine (with about 12% alcohol content)

- 1.5 ounces of distilled spirits or liquor (with about 40% alcohol content)

- **Plan Ahead:** If you know you'll be drinking, plan your meals and snacks to accommodate the extra calories from alcohol. Be mindful of portion sizes and the type of drinks you choose.

- **Choose Wisely:** Opt for lower-calorie and lower-sugar alcoholic beverages. Light beer, dry wines, and spirits with calorie-free mixers are better choices than high-calorie cocktails or sugary drinks.

- **Hydration:** Alternate alcoholic beverages with

water to stay hydrated and help control your overall calorie intake.

- **Limit Frequency:** Avoid frequent alcohol consumption, as it can add up in terms of both calories and potential negative health effects.

- **Track Your Progress:** Keep track of your alcohol consumption and how it fits into your overall dietary plan. Be aware of how it may impact your fat loss progress and adjust accordingly.

CHAPTER 10

HORMONE BALANCE AND FAT LOSS

Hormones play a crucial role in regulating various physiological processes in the body, including metabolism and fat storage. Achieving and maintaining hormone balance is essential for effective fat loss. In this chapter, we'll explore the relationship between hormones and fat loss and provide insights into how to support hormone balance:

1. Insulin:

Insulin is a hormone produced by the pancreas that regulates blood sugar levels. It plays a significant role in fat storage and metabolism.

- **Role in Fat Storage:** High levels of insulin, often seen in individuals with insulin resistance or poor diet choices, can promote fat storage, especially around the abdominal area.

- **Balancing Insulin:** You can help regulate insulin levels by consuming a balanced diet rich in complex carbohydrates, fiber, and lean proteins. Avoid excessive consumption of refined sugars and processed foods.

2. Cortisol:

Cortisol, often referred to as the stress hormone, is produced by the adrenal glands. It plays a role in regulating metabolism and blood sugar levels.

- **Role in Fat Storage:** Chronic stress can lead to elevated cortisol levels, which may promote fat storage, particularly in the abdominal region.

- **Balancing Cortisol:** Strategies for managing stress, such as regular exercise, meditation, deep breathing, and adequate sleep, can help regulate cortisol levels and support fat loss.

3. Lepton:

Lepton is a hormone produced by fat cells that signals to the brain when you're full, helping regulate appetite and energy balance.

- **Role in Fat Loss:** Lepton resistance can occur when the brain becomes less responsive to lepton signals, potentially leading to overeating and weight gain.

- **Balancing Lepton:** Adequate sleep, a balanced diet, and maintaining a healthy weight can help support lepton sensitivity and appetite control.

4. Ghrelin:

Ghrelin is a hormone produced by the stomach that stimulates hunger and appetite.

- **Role in Fat Loss:** Elevated ghrelin levels can increase hunger, potentially leading to overeating and weight gain.

- **Balancing Ghrelin:** Eating regular, balanced meals and snacks throughout the

day can help manage
ghrelin levels and reduce
excessive hunger.

5. Thyroid Hormones:

Thyroid hormones, including
thyroxin (T4) and
triiodothyronine (T3), play a
crucial role in regulating
metabolism.

- **Role in Fat Loss:** An
  underactive thyroid
  (hypothyroidism) can lead
  to a sluggish metabolism

and difficulties with weight management.

. **Balancing Thyroid Hormones:** If you suspect thyroid issues, consult with a healthcare professional for evaluation and potential treatment.

6. Sex Hormones:

Sex hormones, including estrogen and testosterone, play a role in regulating fat storage and metabolism.

- **Role in Fat Loss:** Imbalances in sex hormones can affect fat distribution and muscle mass. For example, low testosterone levels in men can lead to increased fat storage.

- **Balancing Sex Hormones:** Maintaining a healthy weight, regular physical activity, and a balanced diet can support healthy sex hormone levels.

In Summary:

Achieving hormone balance is essential for effective fat loss and overall health. Lifestyle factors such as diet, exercise, stress management, sleep, and maintaining a healthy weight play a significant role in hormone regulation. If you suspect hormonal imbalances are affecting your ability to lose fat or achieve your health goals, consider consulting with a healthcare professional or endocrinologist for evaluation and guidance.

CHAPTER 11

TRACKING YOUR fitness PROGRESS

Tracking your fitness progress is a critical aspect of any fitness journey. It helps you monitor your accomplishments, stay motivated, and make informed adjustments to your exercise and nutrition routines. In this chapter, we'll discuss the importance of tracking fitness progress and provide guidance on how to do it effectively:

1. Set Clear Goals:

Before you start tracking your progress, establish clear and achievable fitness goals. Whether it's losing weight, building muscle, improving endurance, or enhancing flexibility, having specific objectives will guide your tracking efforts.

2. Types of Fitness Progress to Track:

There are various aspects of fitness progress you can track, depending on your goals:

- **Body Measurements:** Regularly measure key areas like waist, hips, chest, arms, and thighs to monitor changes in body composition.

- **Body Weight:** Tracking your weight can provide insights into overall changes, but remember that weight alone doesn't tell the whole story.

- **Strength and Endurance:** Keep a record of your strength training progress by tracking the weight lifted, number of repetitions, and sets. For cardiovascular fitness, note improvements in distance, time, or intensity.

- **Flexibility and Mobility:** Use measurements like the distance you can reach in specific stretches or your performance in mobility exercises to assess improvements.

- **Body Fat Percentage:** If possible, monitor changes in body fat percentage using methods like skinfold caliper, bioelectrical impedance, or DEXA scans.

. **Performance Metrics:** Track specific fitness tests or benchmarks relevant to your goals. For example, monitor the number of push-ups, pull-ups, or your one-rep max in a particular exercise.

3. Choose Tracking Methods:

Select the methods and tools that work best for you in tracking your fitness progress:

- **Fitness Journal:** Maintain a dedicated notebook or digital journal to record your workouts, measurements, and goals.

- **Fitness Apps:** Many apps are available for tracking workouts, nutrition, and progress. They often come with built-in features for setting goals and measuring progress.

- **Progress Photos:** Take regular photos to visually

document changes in your physique. Front, side, and back views are common angles to capture.

. **Wearable Devices:** Wearable fitness trackers and smart watches can record various metrics, including steps, heart rate, and calorie expenditure.

4. Set a Tracking Schedule:

Establish a routine for tracking your progress. Depending on your goals, you may choose to track weekly, biweekly, or monthly. Consistency in tracking is key to seeing meaningful trends.

5. Analyze and Adjust:

Regularly review your tracking data to assess your progress. Use this information to adjust your fitness and nutrition strategies as needed. If you're not seeing the desired results, consider consulting with a fitness professional or trainer for guidance.

6. Celebrate Achievements:

Acknowledge and celebrate your fitness milestones, no matter how small. Recognizing your progress can boost motivation and reinforce positive habits.

7. Stay Patient and Realistic:

Understand that progress may not always be linear, and there will be plateaus and setbacks along the way. Stay patient, stay consistent, and focus on long-term improvements.

8. Listen to Your Body:

While tracking is essential, also pay attention to how your body feels. Rest, recovery, and injury prevention should be prioritized along with progress tracking.

In Summary:

Tracking your fitness progress is a valuable tool for achieving your fitness goals and maintaining motivation. Choose the tracking methods that work best for you, set clear goals, and regularly review your progress. Remember that fitness is a journey, and consistent tracking, along with smart adjustments, will help you stay on the path to success.

CHAPTER 12

FUTURE FITNESS GOAL

Setting future fitness goals is a crucial step in maintaining long-term health and well-being. As you achieve your current goals, it's essential to plan for what comes next to keep your fitness journey exciting and sustainable. In this chapter, we'll explore the importance of setting future fitness goals and provide guidance on how to do it effectively:

1. The Importance of Future Fitness Goals:

Setting future fitness goals serves several important purposes:

- **Maintaining Motivation:** Goals provide a sense of purpose and motivation for your fitness journey. They give you something to work toward and look forward to achieving.

- **Progression:** Goals help you progress and continue

improving your fitness level. Without new challenges, you may plateau or lose interest.

- **Adaptation:** As you achieve current goals, your fitness needs and interests may evolve. Future goals allow you to adapt to these changes.

2. How to Set Future Fitness Goals:

When setting future fitness goals, follow these steps:

- **Reflect on Your Current Goals:** Consider your current fitness goals and accomplishments. Reflect on what you've learned and how your priorities have changed.

- **Identify New Interests:** Explore new fitness activities or disciplines that interest you. This could include trying a new sport, exercise class, or training style.

- **Assess Your Progress:** Evaluate your strengths and weaknesses to identify areas where you want to improve. Whether it's strength, flexibility, endurance, or something else, pinpoints what you'd like to work on.

- **Make Your Goals Specific:** Create clear and specific goals that are measurable. For example, instead of a vague goal like "get in shape," set a specific goal like "run a half marathon in six months."

- **Set Realistic and Achievable Goals:** While it's great to challenge yourself, ensure that your goals are realistic and attainable. Unrealistic goals can lead to frustration and burnout.

- **Create a Timeline:** Establish a timeframe for achieving your future fitness goals.

This provides structure and urgency to your efforts.

- **Break Goals Down:** If your goal is significant, break it down into smaller, manageable milestones. This makes it easier to track progress and stay motivated.

- **Write Down Your Goals:** Document your future fitness goals in writing. This helps solidify your commitment and serves as a reminder.

3. Examples of Future Fitness Goals:

Your future fitness goals can be diverse and tailored to your interests. Here are some examples to consider:

- Running: Participate in a marathon, achieve a specific 5K or 10K time, or complete an obstacle course race.

- Strength Training: Increase your one-rep max in a specific lift, such as the bench press or deadlift.

- Flexibility and Mobility: Master a new yoga pose, improve your range of motion, or achieve a full split.

- Sports: Join a sports league, improve your performance in a particular sport, or learn a new sport or skill like rock climbing or martial arts.

. Weight Management: Reach a specific body composition goal, such as reducing body fat percentage or gaining lean muscle mass.

4. Stay Adaptable:

Remember that your future fitness goals can evolve as you progress. Be adaptable and open to adjusting your goals if your interests or circumstances change. The key is to keep your fitness journey exciting and aligned with your evolving needs and aspirations.

In Summary:

Setting future fitness goals is a vital part of your long-term health and fitness journey. Reflect on your current goals, identify new interests, and create clear and achievable objectives. Your future goals will keep you motivated, help you progress, and ensure that your fitness journey remains fulfilling and enjoyable.

Conclusion

In the final chapters of "Obesity to Fit," we see the culmination of the characters' remarkable journeys. They have traveled a path filled with challenges, victories, and self-discovery, and now it's time to reflect on their transformation.

As we stand at the threshold of this story's conclusion, we witness the characters not only achieving their physical fitness goals but also experiencing profound changes in their lives. Relationships have blossomed, self-esteem has soared, and a newfound sense of purpose permeates their existence.

But the true beauty of this tale lies not just in the pounds shed or muscles gained, but in the lessons learned along the way.

Through their experiences, we come to understand the importance of perseverance, self-compassion, and the unwavering belief in the possibility of change.

"Obesity to Fit" is not just a story about weight loss and physical transformation; it's a testament to the human spirit's resilience. It reminds us that change is possible for anyone who is willing to take the first step, to confront their obstacles head-on, and to embrace the support of loved ones and professionals.

In this conclusion, we also acknowledge that the journey from obesity to fitness is not a linear one. It's marked by setbacks, moments of doubt, and the occasional stumble. But it's precisely these challenges that make the ultimate triumphs all the more remarkable.

As we bid farewell to the characters we've grown to admire and respect, we are left with a sense of hope and inspiration. Their stories serve as a beacon for anyone who may be facing a similar struggle, illuminating the path toward a healthier, happier, and more fulfilling life.

In the end, "Obesity to Fit" leaves us with a profound understanding: transformation is not about reaching a destination; it's about the evolution of the self. It's about discovering the strength within, embracing change, and, most importantly, recognizing that every individual has the power to rewrite their own story, no matter where they start.